REMEDY

If you are sad, read this

GERALD B.K

Introduction

Why this book?

There are moments in life when everything seems to lose its brilliance. Where sadness, like a wave, settles in us, sometimes without warning, sometimes following painful events. It is at these times that we often feel alone, even in the midst of others. If you read this book today, it may be that you are going through one of these periods. Maybe you are looking for comfort, a light to illuminate you in the middle of this tunnel of melancholy. This book was written for you, for those moments when the weight of sadness seems too heavy to you to carry.

The purpose of this book is not to tell you that everything will get better all of a sudden, nor to give you a miracle solution to your sadness. It would be lying to you, and that's not what you deserve. This book is here to accompany you in this process, to show you that even in the darkest moments, it is possible to find a spark of light, a hope that helps you move forward. It is possible to get better, not always in the blink of an eye, but by taking one step after another.

Sadness, a universal emotion

The first thing you need to know is that you are not alone in your sadness. Even if, at the moment, you feel isolated, disconnected from the rest of the world, know that sadness is part of the human condition. Everyone, at one time or another in their life, has felt what you feel. Sadness is a universal emotion, whether you are rich or poor, young or old, in one country or another. It is a natural reaction to certain circumstances: loss, disappointment, uncertainty, or sometimes even a set of small things that accumulate until they form a weight too heavy to carry.

Accepting that sadness is part of life is already a first step towards healing. Sadness allows us to understand the value of moments of happiness. Without the rain, the sun would be just a simple routine, with no particular flavor. What you feel today is part of your journey, and even if it seems insurmountable, you will come out stronger.

Understand that sadness is temporary

When you are immersed in sadness, it is easy to believe that this state will last forever. Emotional pain has this ability to shrink our vision, to make us think that nothing will ever change. But in reality, sadness is temporary. What you feel today will not be what you will feel forever. Emotions are states of passage, even if sometimes they last longer than we would like.

This book is here to help you get through this period, to remind you that sadness is only part of your story, not its entirety. There will be better days, even if you can't imagine them yet.

A personal path to well-being

Each chapter of this book will accompany you on an inner journey. It is not about jumping from one emotion to another by forcing a smile, but rather to offer yourself tools to better understand how you feel, to welcome your emotions without being overwhelmed. The path to emotional well-being is not linear. Sometimes, you will take steps forward, sometimes you will feel like you are retreating. But every little effort counts.

What you will find in this book

Here's what this book offers you:

- Accept your emotions: Sadness is neither good nor bad, it is. Learning to accept it is already defusing part of it.

- Understand the source of your feelings: We will explore together where your sadness comes from, what events or thoughts have nourished it.

- Express your emotions: Whether through speech, writing or other forms of expression, you will discover ways to evacuate this sadness to no longer keep it in you.

- Regain a taste for little things: Even in the heart of sadness, moments of sweetness exist. This book will help you recognize them and cling to them.

- Take care of yourself: Because mind and body are intimately linked, you will discover tips to take care of your physical well-being to support your emotional state.

- Let go and move forward: We will talk about the process of letting go, turning the page, and freeing yourself from the weights that prevent you from moving forward.

A book to read at your own pace

This book is a companion. He won't judge you if you feel sad today and happy tomorrow. He won't force you to get better at a certain speed. You can read it in one go or only a few pages a day, when you feel the need. It is a space for you, a refuge where you can return every time you feel overwhelmed by your emotions.

You are not alone

Maybe this book won't be able to erase your sadness, and that's not its goal. But he will be able, I hope, to remind you that you are not alone, that what you feel is legitimate, and that you have the strength necessary to get through this difficult period. We are all able to overcome our dark moments, even if sometimes it takes time. And even if the road is long, you don't have to travel it alone.

At each stage of this book, remember that sadness is a temporary emotion, that you have the right to feel it, but also the right to let it go. This journey is yours, and you are its hero or heroine. You have the power to move forward, one day after another.

Thus, this book will be your ally, a little guide to accompany you on this journey towards well-being. Together, we will explore what sadness has to teach us, and above all, how to gradually find the light.

Forward for this inner journey!

Chapter 1: Accepting sadness

The first step to overcome sadness is paradoxically to accept it. This may seem counterintuitive. After all, who really wants to be overwhelmed by such a heavy emotion? However, refusing to accept one's emotions can prolong the suffering. In this chapter, we will explore why it is crucial not to fight sadness, but rather to recognize it and accept it as an integral part of life.

1.1. False positivity: Why forcing yourself to be happy can aggravate sadness

In my music album entitled karma as well as in the book of the same title that I recently published. I have always encouraged to stay positive. But this does not mean rejecting sadness, but rather believing that sadness is a temporary feeling. That we must be positive and move forward. But not to force yourself to be happy.

In our modern society, we often value the idea of being constantly positive. We are encouraged to "keep smiling" or "think about something else" when sadness strikes. Social networks are full of images of happiness, success, perfect moments. All this contributes to the pressure of having to be happy, even when it is not our natural state at this precise moment.

But the danger of this approach is that it denies the legitimacy of your emotions. Forcing yourself to be happy when you are not can aggravate sadness. It's like trying to put a bandage on a wound without treating it. The more you ignore your emotions, the more they take up space and seek to express themselves more intensely.

1.2. Acceptance, a path to healing

Accepting sadness is not letting it overwhelm you or immobilize you. It simply means recognizing its existence. Accept that you feel bad and that it is normal to feel this way in certain circumstances. Acceptance is not synonymous with resignation. On the contrary, it is the first step towards a lasting healing.

When you accept to be sad, you stop fighting against yourself. You recognize that sadness is part of the range of human emotions and that you are no less strong because you feel it. Allowing yourself to be sad is showing kindness towards yourself.

> Example : Imagine that sadness is like a rough sea. If you fight the waves, they will overwhelm you. But if you let yourself float, if you accept that the sea is sometimes rough, you can learn to let yourself be carried by the waves rather than drowning.

1.3. Why running away from your emotions is counterproductive

It is natural to want to escape the pain. Often, we try to escape our emotions by occupying the mind with other things: by working too much, spending hours in front of screens or looking for temporary distractions. Yet all these strategies only push back the problem.

Running away from your emotions may seem effective at the moment, but it's like sweeping the dust under the carpet. In the long run, the emotions we repress always end up coming to the surface, sometimes with even more force. This is why it is essential not to turn away from what you feel, even if it seems painful.

> Example : Think of a ball that you are trying to keep under water. The more you put in the force to keep it submerged, the more abruptly it will end up rising to the surface. It's the same with repressed emotions: the more you force them to disappear, the more intensely they will return.

1.4. How to accept your emotions

Accepting emotions is a process that requires practice. Here are some strategies that can help you accommodate your sadness:

Take a moment to recognize it

When you feel the sadness rising in you, stop for a moment. Take a deep breath and be aware of how you feel. Put words on your emotions: "I feel sad. It's normal to feel that. It doesn't define who I am, but it's an emotion present right now."

Don't judge yourself

It is important not to judge yourself for how you feel. Sadness is not a sign of weakness or personal failure. It's a natural emotion. Sadness is often associated with a lack of control or an inability to be happy, but this is not the case. You have the right to feel what you feel.

Create a space for emotion

Giving time to your sadness is a way to accept it. This can be by taking a moment in the day to let you fully feel your emotions, whether by listening to music that touches you, writing what you feel, or simply giving yourself a moment of solitude to reflect.

1.5. Compassion for yourself: being your own friend

Accepting sadness also means showing compassion for yourself. Imagine how you would react if a friend came to see you in tears. You probably wouldn't tell him to "get himself together" or "think about something else". On the contrary, you would listen to him, you would offer him your support, you would tell him that it is normal to be sad sometimes. Why not treat yourself with the same kindness?

> Example : When you feel sad, take a moment to say to yourself: "I'm going

through a difficult time, but it's normal. I will take care of myself as I would for a close friend. I'm not in a hurry to get better, I give myself time."

Compassion for yourself is a key to accepting your emotions. It is to recognize that you are doing your best in a difficult situation and that you deserve to be treated with gentleness and respect, even by yourself.

1.6. The benefits of acceptance

When you accept your sadness, you open the door to several positive things:

A decrease in the intensity of emotions
Curiously, accepting sadness can reduce its intensity. When you stop fighting against her, she loses her power. Sadness then becomes an emotion that you feel, but that does not overwhelm you.

Greater mental clarity

By accepting what you feel, you release the mental energy you used to fight your emotions. This allows you to better understand the situation, identify the root causes of your sadness and consider clearer solutions to get better.

An opening to healing

When you accept your sadness, you put yourself in a position of openness. Rather than remain in denial or struggle, you give yourself the opportunity to heal gently. This can be a slow process, but it is more sustainable.

1.7. Small gestures to accept on a daily basis

Here are some concrete gestures that you can integrate into your daily life to promote the acceptance of your emotions:

- Practice mindfulness

Mindfulness is a technique that consists of being present at the moment, without judgment. When you feel sad, try to focus on your breath, on your physical sensations, and accept your thoughts without trying to change them. Mindfulness can help you welcome your sadness without judging it.

Write your thoughts and emotions

Keeping a diary is a great way to release your emotions. By putting words on what you feel, you make your sadness more tangible and easier to understand. It also allows you to follow your emotional journey over time.

Share with a trusted person

Sometimes, just talking about how you feel can be enough to lighten the weight of sadness. Find a person you trust, someone who can listen to you without judgment, and express your feelings to him.

In conclusion of this chapter, accepting sadness is not easy, but it is an essential step to regain emotional balance. This first step towards acceptance is actually a gesture of love for oneself. Rather than fighting against natural emotions, you learn to welcome them, understand them, and especially let them follow their course without overwhelming you. It is a benevolent approach that will accompany you on your journey towards well-being.

By accepting sadness, you open the door to the possibility of healing, better understanding yourself, and fully living all facets of life, even the darkest, knowing that they will not last forever.

Chapter 2: Understanding the source of his sadness

In this second chapter, we will explore a crucial step on the path to emotional healing: understanding why you feel sad. Sadness, like all emotion, has a reason to be. She does not appear without a cause. Sometimes it stems from obvious events or circumstances. Other times it seems to arise without explanation, but there is always an underlying reason. Understanding where this sadness comes from allows you to demystify it and start working on the root causes to get better.

2.1. The obvious causes and the root causes

Some causes of sadness are easy to identify: a breakup, the loss of a job, the death of a loved one, an argument with a friend. These are external events that have a direct impact on your emotional state. When these events occur, sadness is a natural response. It reflects your pain in the face of loss or disappointment.

But sometimes the causes of sadness are more subtle. You can feel sad without knowing exactly why. This can be due to a set of small frustrations that accumulate, or to deeper and more unconscious causes. Perhaps this sadness comes from something older, from an unexpressed fear, from an inner dissatisfaction. This is why it is essential to examine your emotions closely, in order to understand their origin.

> Example: You can feel sad after a long day of work without having suffered a particular event. However, by thinking about it, you realize that you have been exhausted for several weeks, that you feel devalued by your hierarchy, or that you feel that you lack meaning in what you do. This sadness is therefore the result of an accumulated malaise.

2.2. The weight of unrealised expectations

One of the frequent sources of sadness is the difference between what we hoped for and what we actually get. When our expectations are not met, it creates frustration that can lead to sadness. These expectations can be diverse: they can concern your relationships, your career, your personal ambitions, or even your vision of yourself.

- Expectations of others: Sometimes we expect behaviors or attitudes from others that they cannot or do not want to offer us. This can create a disappointment, especially if we have put a lot of hope in this relationship.

- Expectations of oneself: In the same way, we often set ourselves high goals, and when we fail to achieve them, we feel sadness. This sadness comes from the feeling of failure or devaluation.

> Example : You were hoping for a promotion at work, but it was given to someone else. Your sadness is not only related to this event, but to the accumulation of your broken expectations, the effort made and the feeling of injustice or failure you feel.

2.3. Sadness and the unresolved past

Sadness can also be linked to past wounds that have not been healed. It can be a loss, betrayal, regret or old pain that you have not completely overcome. Sometimes, current events reactivate those old wounds, reviving buried emotions. It is important to ask the question: is this sadness related to a current situation or does it awaken past pain?

> Example : If a romantic relationship ends abruptly and you feel intense sadness, it may be due to the current

breakup, but also to unresolved pain from a previous relationship, or even fears of abandonment rooted in childhood.

Taking the time to think about the links between your past and your present emotions can help you better understand why certain situations affect you more deeply.

2.4. Invisible causes: the role of brain chemistry and external circumstances

Sometimes, sadness does not have an immediate emotional origin, but it is influenced by biological or environmental factors. Lack of sleep, hormonal imbalance, unbalanced diet or physical exhaustion can alter your state of mind and make you more vulnerable to sadness. It is therefore essential to take into account your overall health when you try to understand your sadness.

- Fatigue and stress: Chronic fatigue and prolonged stress can trigger feelings of sadness, even if nothing in your life seems to explain it directly.

- Diet and exercise: A lack of physical exercise or poor diet can also affect your mood. Body and mind are intimately linked, and what you do for your body has an impact on your emotions.

- Climate and seasons: Some people are sensitive to seasonal changes, such as seasonal affective disorder (SAS), where the lack of natural light in winter can cause sadness or depression.

> Example : If you have been feeling sad for a few weeks, it could be related to an accumulation of stress at work, lack of sleep or an unbalanced diet. This kind of sadness doesn't necessarily have a deep emotional cause, but it can be solved by taking care of your body and your physical needs.

2.5. Identify the cause: practical tools

To better understand the source of your sadness, here are some concrete tools that can help you take stock of your emotions:

Reflective writing

Writing is a great way to explore your emotions. Take a notebook or a sheet of paper and start writing freely on how you feel. Don't censor yourself, let the words flow, even if all this seems confusing to you at first. By putting words on your emotions, you will get closer to the source of your sadness.

> Writing exercise: Write on the following questions:

- "What makes me sad right now?"

- "Is there a specific event or situation that triggered this sadness?"

- "Does this sadness remind me of another period of my life?"

2. The observation of emotional patterns

Sometimes our emotions follow recurring patterns. When you feel sad, try to think about past moments when you felt a similar sadness. Does this happen after certain types of events? Is it related to specific expectations you have towards yourself or others?

> Diagram exercise: Try to identify patterns in your emotions. Note the moments when you feel sad and try to see if specific situations or recurring thoughts are at the origin of these feelings.

3. The inner dialogue

Much of the sadness sometimes comes from our own inner dialogue. It is the thoughts that we constantly repeat in our minds that influence our emotions. For example, if you constantly repeat to yourself that you are not up to it, that you are not loved, or that you will never succeed, it can feed your sadness.

> Inner dialogue exercise: Take a few minutes to observe the thoughts that accompany your sadness. Do you criticize yourself or blame yourself excessively? If so, try to reformulate these thoughts in a more benevolent way.

2.6. Learn to be honest with yourself

Understanding the source of your sadness requires emotional honesty. This means being ready to explore aspects of yourself or your life that can be uncomfortable. Maybe your sadness is related to a situation that you don't want to change, like a job or a relationship that makes you unhappy. It is often easier to look away or ignore these sources of sadness, but in the long run, this will only make the situation worse.

> Example: You feel sad every Sunday night at the idea of returning to work on Monday morning. By exploring this, you realize that your work does not satisfy you, but you are afraid of changing careers or looking for another job. The sadness here is a signal that something is wrong, and it encourages you to explore the necessary changes.

2.7. Listen to the signals of your body and mind

Your body and mind are valuable allies in understanding your emotions. Sometimes your body gives you clues about what's going on inside. Sadness can be manifested by unusual fatigue, muscle tension, lack of energy, or sleep disorders. By listening to your body and taking care of it, you will also be able to better understand how you feel.

In the same way, your mind sends you signals. Recurrent thoughts, dreams or even compulsive distractions can be clues about what makes you sad.

Understanding the source of your sadness is a key step to get better. Sadness, whether related to current or past events, disappointed expectations or biological causes, always has a reason for being. By exploring your emotions, identifying the root causes, and being honest with yourself, you can begin to defuse sadness and get closer to a state of well-being.

Chapter 3: The Power of Gratitude and Realistic Positivity

After accepting your sadness and understanding its causes, it's time to change your perspective. In this chapter, we will discuss a powerful and accessible tool to improve your state of mind: gratitude. Many people think that gratitude is just a simplistic concept, but it has a significant impact on how you perceive your life. It is not about ignoring difficulties, but balancing negative thoughts with more conscious attention to the positive aspects of your life.

3.1. What is gratitude?

Gratitude is about recognizing and appreciating the good things that exist in your life, even when it is difficult. It is not a flight from reality or a denial of your problems, but a way to readjust your perception to include the positive aspects that you could neglect by being overwhelmed by sadness.

> Example: Let's imagine that you are going through a difficult period on a personal or professional level. Sadness can make you blind to everything else. But if you take a moment to think about what you appreciate – for example, a loyal friend, a roof over your head, or even a soothing sunset – you redirect your mind to something more positive and feel temporary relief.

3.2. Why is gratitude an antidote to sadness?

Sadness tends to restrict your field of vision. It makes you focus on what is missing, what is wrong, what you have lost. Gratitude, for its part, broadens this field by making you notice what you already have and that works well. It's a powerful emotional rebalancing. Rather than minimizing your feelings, she helps you put your problems into perspective by showing you that not everything is dark.

Here's why gratitude works as an antidote to sadness:

- It reconnects you to the present moment: Gratitude brings you back to the moment. Rather than rehashing the past or anticipating the future, you focus on what is good here and now.

It modifies brain chemistry: Studies have shown that it regularly practices active gratitude in areas of the brain associated with positive emotions and well-being. This lowers levels of stress and anxiety.

- It changes your perspective: Gratitude encourages you to see life from a more balanced angle. Rather than focusing only on what makes you sad, it allows you to appreciate the little positive things that you can often forget.

3.3. Realistic positivity vs blind optimism

Practicing gratitude and cultivating a positive attitude does not mean ignoring problems or pretending that everything is fine. It is essential to differentiate between realistic positivity and blind optimism.

- Blind optimism: It is ignoring reality, refusing to see the problems, and pretending that everything is fine when it is not. This can lead to an accumulation of frustration and repressed emotions.

- Realistic positivity: It is recognizing that life has ups and downs, but choosing to also focus on the positive aspects, without denying the difficulties. This allows you to maintain an emotional balance and face problems with more resilience.

> Example: If you are going through a period of grief or breakup, it would be unrealistic to pretend that everything is fine and that you do not feel any pain.

Realistic positivity allows you to recognize your sadness while finding moments of comfort, whether spending time with friends or appreciating an act of kindness.

3.4. How to practice gratitude on a daily basis

It is easy to understand the theory of gratitude, but how to put it into practice in everyday life? Here are some simple and effective techniques to integrate gratitude into your daily life:

The gratitude diary

Take a few minutes every day to write three things you are grateful for. It can be simple things like a good meal, a pleasant conversation, or a stranger's smile. By putting them in writing, you strengthen your attention on these positive moments and create a ritual that leads your mind to look for reasons to feel good.

> Exercise: Every night before going to bed, write down three things you are grateful for during the day, regardless of their size or importance.

2. Meditation of gratitude

Close your eyes and take a few minutes to focus on a person, a memory, or an object for which you feel gratitude. Take a deep breath by visualizing this source of gratitude and feel the positive emotions it arouses in you.

> Exercise : Devote five minutes every morning to meditating on something for which you feel grateful. This can give you good energy to start the day.

3. Express your gratitude

Do not hesitate to express your gratitude to others. Saying "thank you" or showing appreciation to someone can not only strengthen your relationships, but also strengthen your own sense of well-being.

The more you share gratitude, the more gratitude you feel.

> Exercise : Every week, take the time to send a message or tell someone in your life what you like about him or her.

4. Look for the positive aspects in the difficulties

Even in difficult times, it is possible to find something to be grateful for. For example, a test may have made you stronger, or a complicated situation may have allowed you to learn an important lesson. Practicing this form of gratitude can help you change your perception of negative events.

> Example: After a test, ask yourself: "What did this situation teach me? How do I grow up?"

3.5. Reconfigure your mind for positivity

Our brain has a natural tendency to focus on the negative, what psychologists call the "negativity bias". This bias pushes us to give more weight to negative experiences than to positive experiences. The good news is that you can train your brain to reverse this pattern.

Gratitude and realistic positivity act as a mental exercise. The more you practice them, the more you strengthen your ability to see the positive in your life. Over time, it becomes a habit. When you reorient your mind towards positivity, you become more resilient to life's challenges and reduce your feeling of sadness.

- Take a step back: When you face a difficulty, try to take a step back. Ask yourself the question: "What is the positive part in this situation?" Even in the darkest situations, there are often lessons to be learned or moments of light that can emerge.

- Change your inner dialogue: Replace negative thoughts with more balanced affirmations. For example, instead of telling yourself "I'll never make it," try to tell yourself "It's hard, but I do my best and I learn along the way."

> Exercise : The next time you feel overwhelmed by sadness, take a break and find at least one positive thing in your day, no matter how small it is. It can be something as simple as taking a break for you, or meeting someone who smiled at you.

3.6. The benefits of gratitude in the long term

The benefits of gratitude and realistic positivity are not limited to immediate relief. In the long term, they improve your overall well-being. Here are some of the long-term benefits:

Stress reduction: Gratitude lowers levels of cortisol, the stress hormone, which helps you feel calmer and more relaxed.

Improved mental health: Regularly practicing gratitude is linked to a decrease in symptoms of depression and an increase in positive emotions.

Better social relationships: When you express your gratitude to others, you strengthen your social ties, which improves your emotional support.

- Strengthening resilience: By cultivating a positive and realistic attitude, you become more resistant to the trials of life. This allows you to better manage difficult moments without being overwhelmed by sadness.

3.7. The limits of gratitude: when accepting it is not enough

It is important to note that gratitude, although powerful, is not a miracle solution. Sometimes the sadness or depression is too deep to be soothed by the sole practice of gratitude. If you find yourself in a situation where your emotions are too heavy to manage alone, it is essential not to hesitate to ask for professional help.

Gratitude and realistic positivity are not instant responses to sadness, but powerful tools that can help you reorient your mind towards more positive aspects of your life. By learning to recognize the small blessings that surround you and developing a balanced state of mind, you strengthen your ability to go through difficult times with more resilience and serenity. These practices allow you to rediscover the beauty of everyday life, even when everything seems dark.

Chapter 4: Reconnecting to yourself through self-compassion

In this chapter, we will explore the importance of self-compassion, an essential key to overcoming sadness. If gratitude helps us recognize the positive aspects of life, self-compassion helps us recognize and accept our humanity, our vulnerability, and our imperfections. Reconnecting to yourself through self-compassion is learning to be benevolent towards yourself, even in moments of pain and sadness.

4.1. What is self-compassion?

Self-compassion is the ability to offer yourself the same kindness and understanding that you would offer to a close friend. While most people are naturally compassionate towards others, they are often hard on themselves, judging themselves severely when they are sad, disappointed or fail.

Self-compassion involves three key elements:

Kindness towards yourself: Be gentle with yourself when you suffer, instead of criticizing or judging yourself severely.

The sense of common humanity: Recognizing that suffering and imperfection are human experiences shared by all. You are not alone in your sadness.

- Mindfulness: Observe your emotions with clarity and without judgment, instead of repressing them or letting yourself be overwhelmed by them.

Self-compassion allows you to treat yourself with understanding and empathy in moments of sadness, instead of aggravating your suffering with negative internal criticism.

> Example : If you're going through a difficult time after a failure or a breakup, instead of saying to yourself "I suck, I didn't deserve to succeed", self-compassion invites you to recognize your pain by saying "It's hard right now, but I'm doing my best and I have the right to feel it."

4.2. Why is it so difficult to be compassionate towards yourself?

Many people find it easy to support others, but are very critical of themselves. This attitude often comes from ingrained beliefs about how to succeed or "do things well".

The belief that criticism motivates us: Many think that self-criticizing pushes them to do better. "If I'm hard on myself, I'll improve." But in reality, excessive internal criticism fuels doubt, fear of failure, and sadness.

The fear of becoming complacent: Some fear that if they are too kind to themselves, they will become lazy or complacent. They confuse self-compassion with permissiveness or complacency.

- Social standards: Society often values success, productivity, and strength. As a result, it is easy to feel inadequate if you do not meet these expectations. This leads to self-criticism rather than self-compassion.

> Example : You may have grown up in an environment where excellence and perfection were highly valued. In case of failure or difficulty, you have learned to criticize yourself to improve. However, this approach can become toxic and fuel a circle of negativity, making sadness more difficult to overcome.

4.3. The impact of self-compassion on sadness

Self-compassion has a profound effect on the way you deal with sadness and suffering. Rather than seeing sadness as a sign of weakness or failure, self-compassion allows you to accept it as a normal part of the human experience.

Here's how self-compassion can ease sadness:

- Reduction of negative judgments: Self-compassion replaces internal criticism with comforting words. This reduces the intensity of negative emotions and the tendency to blame yourself.

Emotional regulation: When you are benevolent towards yourself, you soothe your emotions, which helps you better regulate them and prevent them from becoming overwhelming.

- Reduction of isolation: By recognizing that others also share moments of sadness, you feel less isolated in your suffering. This creates a sense of connection, which can lighten your sadness.

> Example : If you fail an important project, self-compassion allows you to recognize your disappointment without judging yourself severely. You say to yourself "It's normal to feel sad, but I'll get over it. It's not a total failure, I learned something."

4.4. Practice self-compassion on a daily basis

Like any skill, self-compassion requires practice. Here are some ways to integrate it into your daily life:

Talk to yourself with kindness

Start by observing your inner dialogue. When you find yourself criticizing yourself, imagine what you would say to a friend in the same situation, and tell yourself. Replace harsh words with words of comfort and encouragement.

> Exercise : Every time you criticize yourself, take a moment to reformulate this thought with kindness. For example, replace "I'll never make it" with "It's hard, but I can do it if I keep trying."

2. Recognizing common humanity

Remember that you are not alone in feeling sadness. All humans go through difficult times. By recognizing that suffering is part of human experience, you reduce the feeling of isolation that often accompanies sadness.

> Exercise: When you feel sad, remember: "Other people feel the same thing right now. I'm not alone."

3. Practice mindfulness

Mindfulness helps you to be attentive to your emotions without judging them. It means observing your thoughts and feelings without trying to flee or change them. By being fully aware of your sadness, you can understand and manage it more effectively.

> Exercise : When you feel sad, sit quietly and take a few deep breaths. Notice where the sadness is in your body (chest, stomach, etc.).

Breathe in this area without trying to get rid of the sensation. Just watch her.

4. Self-soothing gestures

Sometimes a simple gesture can ease your emotional pain. It can be putting your hand on your heart, wrapping yourself in a blanket or taking a hot bath. These self-appeasement gestures remind you that you deserve comfort.

> Exercise : Whenever you feel overwhelmed by sadness, take a moment to make a gesture that brings you physical comfort, such as a hug to yourself or a comforting cup of tea.

4.5. Self-compassion and responsibility

Self-compassion is not an excuse to escape one's responsibilities or ignore one's mistakes. On the contrary, it allows you to face your mistakes with more clarity and courage. When you treat yourself with compassion, you are more inclined to recognize your weaknesses and work to improve them, without feeling crushed by guilt.

Self-compassion encourages you to ask yourself: "How can I learn from this experience?" Instead of telling you "I'm a loser." It pushes you to grow and evolve, while being gentle/sweet with yourself.

4.6. The power of forgiveness towards oneself

An essential part of self-compassion is forgiveness towards oneself. We all make mistakes, but it is often easier to forgive others than ourselves. Self-forgiving does not mean ignoring your mistakes, but rather accepting that you did your best at that time with the resources at your disposal.

Forgiveness to yourself frees you from chains of regret and guilt, which can be deep sources of sadness.

> Example : If you have made a bad decision in the past that still haunts you, practicing self-compassion consists of recognizing that, even if you have made a mistake, it does not define you. Forgive yourself for this mistake, and use it as a lesson to move forward.

4.7. The long-term benefits of self-compassion

Practicing self-compassion in the long term transforms your relationship with yourself and with others. Here are some of the benefits:

- Reduction of anxiety and depression: Self-compassion is linked to a decrease in anxiety, depression and shame.

-Improved resilience: Self-compassionate people are more resilient to life's trials. They get up faster after a fall.
- Strengthening self-esteem: Self-compassion allows you to develop self-esteem that is not based on your successes or failures, but on unconditional acceptance of yourself.

Reconnecting to yourself through self-compassion is a crucial step in overcoming sadness. By learning to treat yourself with kindness, to accept your imperfections, and to forgive your mistakes, you create an inner space where sadness can be welcomed without judgment. This approach allows you to go through difficult times with more gentleness and resilience, and to emerge stronger and more serene.

Chapter 5: The power of relationships and social support

In moments of sadness, it is easy to withdraw into yourself and cut yourself off from the world. Yet social support is one of the most powerful factors in regaining joy and hope. In this chapter, we will explore how relationships – whether friendly, family or community – play a crucial role in the emotional healing process. We will also discuss how to create, nurture and strengthen these bonds to make the most of them in times of sadness.

5.1. The importance of social support for emotional well-being

Human beings are social creatures by nature. Our ancestors have always survived in groups, and our brain is wired to create and maintain connections.

Social support is not just a bonus for emotional life, it is a basic need. Studies have shown that people who maintain strong social relationships are generally happier, live longer and have better mental health.

When you feel sad, turning to others can help you share your burden, receive comfort and feel less alone. Friends, family or even members of a community can provide encouragement, different perspectives, and a space to express your emotions without judgment.

> Example: After a difficult breakup, talking to a close friend or a member of your family can bring you comfort. Sharing your thoughts and emotions, even if you don't have all the answers, gives you the opportunity to get out of isolation and see the situation from a different angle.

5.2. The different types of social support

There are several types of social support, and each plays a different role in your emotional life. By understanding the different forms of support, you can learn to identify what you need at a given time, and to seek that support proactively.

Emotional support

This type of support is about listening, empathy and encouragement. It often comes from close people, such as friends, partners or family members. Emotional support allows you to feel understood and accepted in your moments of vulnerability. It helps reduce sadness by making you feel that you are not alone in your experience.

> Example : When you have had a difficult day, receiving a message of encouragement from a friend or

discussing your emotions with a loved one allows you to feel seen and heard.

2. Practical or material support

Sometimes, in moments of sadness or difficulty, you need help to accomplish daily tasks. This support can include financial assistance, help with household chores, or simple gestures such as preparing a meal. Receiving this kind of support lightens the burden and allows you to focus on your emotional well-being.

> Example : After losing a job or going through a difficult ordeal, a friend who helps you reorganize your finances or offers to take care of the shopping can have a significant impact on your ability to manage the situation.

3. Informational support

It is a support that consists of giving advice, information or new perspectives. This can come from a mentor, a colleague, or even a therapy. Information support can help you find solutions or strategies to overcome emotional or practical challenges.

> Example : If you are going through grief or a difficult situation, consulting a therapist or reading books on grief can provide you with tools to better understand and navigate this period.

4. Support through belonging

Feeling that you are part of a group or community can be a powerful form of support. Whether it's a religious community, a support group, or a sports team, these groups provide a sense of belonging that can reduce sadness and isolation.

> Example : Joining a support group for people going through an experience similar to yours, such as a talking group for those who are experiencing a breakup, can bring you comfort by connecting with

other people who understand what you are going through.

5.3. Cultivate positive and meaningful relationships

When sadness takes over, it is essential to cultivate and maintain relationships that give you support. However, not all relationships are equal in terms of quality and impact on your well-being. It is therefore important to focus on connections that are healthy, caring and mutual.

1. Surround yourself with benevolent people

Relationships that nourish you emotionally are those that are based on trust, respect and empathy. These people listen to you without judging you, encourage you in difficult times, and offer you a safe space to be yourself. Surrounding yourselves with caring people can make a huge difference in the way you go through sadness.

> Exercise: Identify the people in your life who make you feel listened to and understood. Spend more time with them, and don't hesitate to open up to them when you feel vulnerable.

2. Avoid toxic relationships

Some relationships can, on the contrary, aggravate your sadness. People who criticize you, judge you or minimize your emotions can make your situation harder to manage. These toxic relationships can make you feel even more isolated and misunderstood.

> Example : If a friend regularly tells you "You dramatize too much, it's not so serious", it can minimize your emotions and make you doubt the legitimacy of your sadness. In these cases, it is important to limit these interactions or to distance yourself.

3. Invested in mutual relationships

Balanced relationships are those where support goes both ways. These are not only relationships where you give or receive, but relationships where everyone takes care of the other. Investing in these relationships creates a solid foundation to receive support when you need it, and to offer support in return.

> Example : If a friend listens to you and supports you in your moments of sadness, also be careful to be there for him/her in his/her difficult moments. Reciprocity strengthens the bond and ensures that the relationship is balanced.

5.4. How to ask for help when you feel sad

Many people have trouble asking for help when they are going through a period of sadness. This can be due to the fear of being a burden, shame or the idea of having to appear strong. However, asking for help is an act of courage and a proof of strength, not weakness.

Identify your needs

Before asking for help, take a moment to think about what you really need. Do you need to talk to someone to express your emotions, or more practical help, such as help with daily tasks? Identifying your needs allows you to better formulate your request and be more specific.

2. Express your needs clearly

When you ask for help, be clear and direct. It is often useful to start by expressing how you feel and why you need support. This can facilitate the conversation and help the other person understand your emotional state.

> Example: "I'm going through a difficult time right now, and I really need to talk to someone. Would you have time for us to have a coffee together this week?"

3. Accept that others can't solve everything

Sometimes, even with the best social support, there are times when no one can "solve" the source of your sadness. However, just because they can't fix everything doesn't mean they can't bring you comfort or support. Their presence alone can be enough to lighten your burden.

4. Don't wait until you're at the end of the roll to ask for help

Don't wait to be overwhelmed by your sadness to ask for support. The more proactive you are in your search for help, the easier it will be to go through difficult times before they become too overwhelming.

> Example : Rather than closing in on yourself after a hard blow, take the initiative to contact a friend or relative and plan an outing or activity. This can be

an easy way to reconnect and avoid isolation.

5.5. The role of the community and support groups

In addition to individual relationships, belonging to a wider community can be a priceless source of comfort and healing. Support groups, religious or spiritual communities, and even local associations can offer you opportunities to connect with people sharing similar experiences.

- Support groups: Support groups allow you to share your emotions in a secure space with people who are having similar experiences. Whether it's a support group for grief, depression, or breakup management, these groups offer a framework to express your sadness without judgment.

- Spiritual communities: If you are part of a religious or spiritual community, it can also be a source of comfort and belonging. Shared beliefs and collective practices can strengthen your sense of connection to something greater and help you through difficult times.

Human relationships and social support play a fundamental role in the emotional healing process. By cultivating positive connections, asking for help when you need it, and surrounding yourself with a caring community, you create a strong network to overcome sadness. The strength of relationships lies not only in the ability of others to solve your problems, but in their constant presence and their ability to remind you that you are not alone in your suffering.

Chapter 6: The power of body and mind: integrating movement and mindfulness

In this chapter, we will explore the powerful bond between body and mind, and how physical movement and mindfulness can help relieve sadness and promote lasting emotional healing. Often, when you are sad, you feel stuck mentally and emotionally, as if the energy was no longer flowing freely. The body and mind are intimately linked, and by adopting practices that engage these two aspects, you can gradually get out of this state of stagnation.

6.1. The link between body and mind

Sadness does not reside only in the mind; it is also expressed in the body. It can manifest itself in the form of physical tension, fatigue, muscle pain, digestive problems, or even a general feeling of heaviness. Emotions, positive or negative, have a direct impact on our physical condition.

The body and mind work in an interconnected way: what affects one often has an effect on the other. Thus, by acting on your body through movement, you can influence your mind, and vice versa. The key is to understand that sometimes, to get better mentally, it is necessary to start by acting physically.

> Example: If you feel sad and it makes you want to stay inactive all day, it can be difficult to motivate you to move. However, a simple 10 to 15 minute walk in nature can help change your state of mind by releasing endorphins and soothing the nervous system.

6.2. The impact of the movement on sadness

Physical movement, whether intense or gentle, is one of the most effective methods to improve your mood and reduce sadness. Physical activity stimulates the production of endorphins, hormones of well-being, which act as a natural antidote against depression and anxiety. It also increases the level of serotonin and dopamine, two neurotransmitters that play a key role in mood regulation.

1. The role of endorphins

Endorphins are neurotransmitters produced by the brain in response to physical activity. They have a natural analgesic effect and help reduce physical and emotional pain. After an exercise, even light, you can feel lighter/lighter, less overwhelmed, and more optimistic.

2. Improvement of energy circulation

When you are sad, it is common to feel a stagnation of energy. Movement, even moderate, helps to reactivate the circulation of energy in your body. This allows you to free yourself from the weight of sadness and breathe new life into your mind.

3. Reduction of anxiety

In times of sadness, anxiety can also be present. Regular physical activity helps reduce this anxiety by regulating the heart rate and promoting better stress management. Even a gentle activity such as yoga or walking can have soothing effects.

6.3. Physical practices to calm the mind

There are many forms of movement that can help you calm your mind and transform your energy. The goal is not to practice a high-intensity sport (unless you want to), but rather to find a type of movement that suits you and that is good for you, whether it is an intense or softer activity.

1. Conscious walking

Walking is one of the simplest and most accessible forms of exercise. It can be practiced anywhere and does not require any equipment. Conscious walking is walking slowly paying attention to each step, to your breath, and to your environment. This form of walking combines movement and mindfulness, which allows you to reconnect to your body and calm your mind.

> Example : Take 20 minutes to walk in a park or in a quiet neighborhood. Breathe deeply and be attentive to every sensation in your body: the contact of your feet with the ground, the breeze on your face, the surrounding sounds. This practice helps you reconnect to the present moment and alleviate sadness.

2. Yoga

Yoga is a millennial practice that combines physical movement, breathing and meditation. There are many types of yoga, some more dynamic, others more focused on relaxation. Yoga can be a powerful tool to release the physical tensions related to sadness, calm the mind, and bring a sense of inner peace.

> Example : Try a gentle yoga session, such as hatha yoga or yin yoga, which focus on postures maintained for a long time and deep stretches. These practices promote the relaxation of the body and allow to release the emotions stored in the muscles.

3. The dance

Dance is another expressive and liberating way of moving. It allows you to get out of your head and reconnect to your body in a fun and joyful way. Dance gives you the freedom to express your emotions through movement, without the need to verbalize them.

> Example: Put on your favorite music and let your body move as it wishes. Don't worry about dancing well or following specific movements. Let yourself go and use dance as a way to evacuate tensions and have fun.

6.4. Mindfulness: anchoring in the present moment

Mindfulness is a practice that consists of being fully present in the moment, without judgment. It helps to observe your thoughts and emotions with kindness and without trying to flee them. By cultivating mindfulness, you learn to observe your sadness, not as something to reject, but as an emotion to welcome with curiosity and compassion.

1. The observation of thoughts and emotions

In times of sadness, it is easy to be overwhelmed by negative thoughts. Mindfulness helps you take a step back from these thoughts by simply observing them without clinging to them. You can imagine that these thoughts are like clouds that pass through the sky: they come and go without you has to hold them back.

> Example : When you feel sad, take a few minutes to sit in silence and observe the thoughts that cross your mind. Take a deep breath and visualize these thoughts as clouds. Notice them without judging them or trying to chase them.

2. Conscious breathing

Breathing is a powerful tool to calm the mind and calm the body. Conscious breathing consists of paying special attention to your breath, which helps you refocus and calm the flow of thoughts. It is a simple but very effective practice to reduce sadness and anxiety.

> Example : Sit in a quiet place and focus on your breathing. Inhale deeply by

counting to four, hold your breath for two seconds, then exhale slowly counting to six. Repeat this breath for five to ten minutes. It will help relax your body and calm your mind.

3. Guided meditation

Guided meditation is a form of meditation where you follow a voice or recording that guides you through the process. This can be especially useful if you are new to meditation or if you have trouble concentrating. Guided meditations can help you explore specific themes, such as emotional healing or self-compassion.

> Example : Find a guided meditation focused on emotional healing or managing sadness. Get comfortable and listen to the voice guide you through a series of breathing, visualization and relaxation exercises.

6.5. Combine movement and mindfulness

Combining movement and mindfulness maximizes the benefits on body and mind. When you move consciously, you give your mind a point of concentration while releasing physical tensions. This combination creates a state of "flow" where you are totally present, absorbed by the experience of the moment.

1. Qi gong and tai chi

These Chinese practices combine slow and fluid movements with breathing and mental concentration. They are often considered "meditations in motion". They help balance internal energy, calm the nervous system, and bring inner peace. These practices are particularly effective in releasing sadness stuck in the body while soothing the mind.

> Example : If you feel tired or depressed, try a qi gong or tai chi session.

Gentle and repetitive movements, combined with conscious breathing, help restore emotional balance and relax the body.

2. Yoga in full awareness

When you practice yoga in full awareness, you focus not only on the postures, but also on the quality of your breathing and the state of your mind. This approach makes each movement more intentional and helps you stay anchored in the present moment.

> Example: During your next yoga session, pay special attention to each movement. Breathe deeply at each transition and observe how your body reacts. This practice will help you strengthen the connection between your body and mind.

Movement and mindfulness are two powerful tools to transform sadness and regain a state of well-being. By integrating physical practices adapted to your energy level, and by cultivating mindfulness through breathing and meditation, you promote both physical and emotional healing. The body and mind being deeply linked, by taking care of one, you positively influence the other, thus creating a virtuous circle of well-being and resilience.

Chapter 7: The importance of creativity and personal expression

Creativity is a powerful resource to overcome sadness. It allows you to express complex emotions, find meaning in your experiences and discover aspects of yourself that can be hidden or repressed. In this chapter, we will explore how to integrate creativity into your life to help you through times of sadness, using various forms of personal expression.

7.1. Creativity as a healing tool

Creativity is not only reserved for artists or people with an innate aptitude for drawing, music or writing. It is an inherent ability of all human beings and can be used as a way to treat and understand your emotions. Creative expression allows you to shape what you feel and what you live, often more deeply than words alone allow.

1. The expression of emotions through art

Art is a powerful way to highlight what you feel inside. Whether you are a painter, a designer, or just use a sketchbook, creating art allows you to release your emotions and explore them in a safe space.

> Example : If you feel sad, take a few hours to draw or paint what you feel. Don't worry about the aesthetic quality. The important thing is to focus on the process and give free rein to your personal expression.

2. Music as an emotional refuge

Music is another form of creativity that can deeply touch your mind and heart. Whether you choose to listen to music that resonates with your mood or take an instrument to play or sing, music can be a powerful emotional therapy.

> Example : Create a playlist of songs that comfort you or express what you feel. If you play an instrument, compose a piece or play songs that help you express and understand your emotions.

3. Writing as a tool for reflection and liberation

Writing is a way to put words on your thoughts and feelings. Whether you choose to keep a diary, write poems, or write letters (which you may not send), writing allows you to explore your emotions, outsource them, and sometimes transform them.

> Example : Write a letter to yourself or someone who hurt you, but do not send the letter. Use this writing as a way to release your emotions and find some clarity.

7.2. Discover and nurture your own creativity

Finding your own creative path can be a journey of personal discovery. Each has unique forms of creative expression that resonate with him or her. Here are some steps to help you discover and nurture your own creativity:

1. Exploration of creative interests

Sometimes it is necessary to give yourself permission to explore different forms of creativity to find out what suits you best. Try various creative activities without setting limits or judgments. Painting, writing, music, dance, sculpture, photography, sewing, etc., are all ways to express yourself.

> Example : If you have never tried pottery, sign up for a local workshop or buy a kit for beginners. The important thing is to remain open and curious about the various creative possibilities.

2. Create a space dedicated to creativity

Having a specific space for your creative activities can help you focus and free yourself from distractions. It can be a corner of your apartment, a workshop, or even an office where you keep all your creative materials and tools.

> Example : Arrange a corner of your living space with art supplies, a sketchbook, and a comfortable place to work. This dedicated place will encourage you to spend more time exploring your creativity.

3. Make creativity a regular practice

For creativity to become a real healing tool, it is useful to practice it regularly. Even if it's only a few minutes a day, integrating creative moments into your daily routine can have a significant impact on your emotional well-being.

> Example : Reserve 15 to 30 minutes each day for a creative activity, such as writing in your diary, playing an instrument, or working on an artistic project. Make this practice a ritual that allows you to refocus.

7.3. Creativity in moments of sadness

Sadness can sometimes paralyze creativity, making it difficult to find inspiration or energy to engage in creative activities. However, it is often in these moments that creativity can be the most beneficial. The key is to allow creativity to be a form of liberation rather than an obligation.

1. Use creativity to explore sadness

When you feel sad, use creativity to explore and express that sadness. The creative process can provide you with an outlet for repressed emotions and help you understand and accept what you are going through.

> Example : Create a collage or a series of drawings that visually represent what you feel. Don't try to create something "beautiful" or "perfect"; focus on the process and how it helps you release your emotions.

2. Let sadness guide the creative process

Allow sadness to influence your creative work. Sometimes emotions can guide your art in an unexpected and revealing way. Accept that your creative work can reflect the depth of your sadness and consider it an integral part of the healing process.

> Example : Write a poem or a song inspired by your sadness. Allow yourself to dive deep into your emotions and explore how they translate into your words or melodies.

3. Find comfort in the creative process

Sometimes, the mere fact of engaging in a creative activity can bring temporary relief from sadness. The process itself can be soothing, offering a moment of concentration and calm that contrasts with the state of distress.

> Example : When sadness seems overwhelming, take a moment to draw or paint. Focus on gesture and movement, and allow yourself to find comfort in creating something tangible and personal.

7.4. The art of sharing and celebrating your creativity

Sharing your creative work with others can also be a healing act. This allows you to show a part of yourself, connect with other people, and receive encouragement that can be deeply comforting.

1. Share with friends or a creative community

Join online or in-person groups or communities that share similar creative interests. These groups can offer support, encouragement and a platform to share your creations.

> Example : Share your works of art, writings or musical creations with close friends or on dedicated forums. Positive feedback and community support can provide a sense of validation and belonging.

2. Participate in exhibitions or performances

If you are comfortable, consider participating in local art exhibitions, reading evenings or concerts. These events offer an opportunity to showcase your work and celebrate your creative achievements with an audience.

> Example : Register for a local art exhibition or an open mic evening to share your creations with others. This

experience can be rewarding and give you a sense of pride and accomplishment.

3. Celebrate small victories

Recognizing and celebrating the small steps of your creative process is essential. Whether it's the realization of a project, the discovery of a new technique, or simply taking time to create, every victory is an important step towards healing.

> Example : When you finish a creative project, take a moment to recognize it and celebrate your achievement. Whether by sharing your work with others or rewarding yourself with an activity you enjoy, valuing these moments motivates you to continue creating.

Creativity and personal expression offer a rich and deep way to navigate through sadness. By integrating creative practices into your daily life, you give yourself the tools to explore, understand and transform your emotions. Creativity is not limited to art or music; it is a way of connecting to yourself and the world around you. By cultivating and celebrating your own creativity, you create a space for healing and personal growth, transforming sadness into an opportunity for expression and discovery.

Chapter 8: Finding meaning and gratitude in difficult times

When sadness seems to invade every aspect of your life, it can be difficult to see the light at the end of the tunnel. However, even in the darkest moments, it is possible to find meaning and gratitude. This chapter looks at how to discover the meaning in your trials and cultivate gratitude, two essential aspects to transform sadness into an opportunity for growth and resilience.

8.1. The quest for meaning in the face of sadness

Finding meaning in trials can help you cope with sadness and transcend it. This does not mean that you should minimize or ignore your pain, but rather that you seek to understand and accept what you are going through as part of a broader journey.

1. The prospect of personal growth

Difficult times can be opportunities for personal growth. By reflecting on what you have learned from your experiences and how they have shaped you, you can find a deeper meaning in what you are going through. These experiences can help you develop qualities such as resilience, empathy and inner strength.

> Example : Take a moment to write about the lessons you learned during this difficult period. How have these experiences helped you develop as a person? What new skills or perspectives have you acquired?

2. The search for meaning through passions and values

By reconnecting with your passions and values, you can find meaning in your experiences. This process can include exploring what motivates you deeply and what gives you a sense of accomplishment and satisfaction, even in times of sadness.

> Example : Think about what you are really passionate about and how you can integrate these passions into your daily life. This can include participating in activities that bring you closer to your core values and remind you of what is important to you.

3. The impact of perspective on meaning

The way you choose to perceive challenges can influence your ability to find meaning. Adopting a perspective of curiosity and openness to difficulties can help you see these moments as learning opportunities rather than as insurmountable obstacles.

> Example : When you face a challenge, try to see it as a chance to discover something about yourself or about life. Ask yourself questions such as: "What can

I learn from this situation?" Or "How can I use this experience to grow?"

8.2. Cultivate gratitude in times of sadness

Gratitude is a powerful practice that can transform the way you experience sadness. By focusing on what you are grateful for, you can change your state of mind and cultivate a sense of inner peace, even in the face of adversity.

1. The daily practice of gratitude

Incorporating gratitude into your daily routine can help you maintain a positive outlook. Even in difficult times, taking the time to recognize the little things you are grateful for can bring a more balanced and soothing perspective.

> Example : Every day, write down three things you are grateful for. It can be as simple as a friend's support, a moment of tranquility, or even a personal fulfillment.

Repeating this practice regularly will help you strengthen your sense of gratitude.

2. Writing letters of gratitude

Writing letters of gratitude to people who have had a positive impact on your life can be a powerful way to strengthen your gratitude practice. These letters do not need to be sent; the main thing is to focus on expressing your gratitude.

> Example : Write a letter to someone who supported you during this difficult time. Clearly express what you are grateful for and how this person has made a difference in your life. Even if you don't send it, this gesture will help you recognize and value the positive aspects of your life.

3. Finding gratitude in the little things

Sometimes it's easier to cultivate gratitude by focusing on the little things in everyday life. These small sources of happiness can offer comfort and remind you that, even in times of sadness, there are always positive elements to appreciate.

> Example : Take the time every day to notice and appreciate the little things, such as a hot cup of tea, a smile of a stranger, or a moment of calm. By focusing on these simple aspects, you enrich your perspective and strengthen your sense of gratitude.

8.3. Resilience and inner strength

Finding meaning and cultivating gratitude are important aspects of the path to resilience. Resilience is the ability to bounce back after difficulties, to adapt and to move forward despite challenges. By building your resilience, you strengthen your ability to cope with sadness and come out stronger.

1. Develop a resilient attitude

Adopting a resilient attitude implies seeing challenges as opportunities to grow and strengthen yourself. It means recognizing that difficulties are part of life and that you have the ability to overcome them.

> Example : When you are faced with an obstacle, try to ask yourself how you can use this situation to strengthen yourself. What skills can you develop? What aspects of your life can be improved through this experience?

2. Strategies to strengthen resilience

Resilience can be enhanced by various practices, such as social support, self-compassion, and setting realistic goals. By integrating these strategies into your life, you create a solid foundation to face difficulties.

> Example : Surround yourself with people who encourage and support you. Set achievable goals and celebrate each

small victory. Practice self-compassion by being kind to yourself and recognizing that facing difficulties is a normal part of the journey.

3. The importance of flexibility and acceptance

Resilience also involves flexibility and acceptance. Accepting that certain things are out of your control and being ready to adapt to changing circumstances is essential to maintain a positive and advanced state of mind despite trials.

> Example : If you are facing an unexpected change or a setback, try to remain open to the possibility that this situation could offer new opportunities. Adjust your expectations and plans accordingly, keeping in mind that flexibility can help reduce stress and promote resilience.

8.4. Finding meaning in relationships and contributions

Relationships and contributions to others can also provide a deep meaning and strengthen your sense of gratitude. Helping others and creating meaningful connections can bring a new perspective and enrich your experience.

1. Engage in altruistic actions

Helping others can offer a meaning and satisfaction that goes beyond one's own concerns. Altruistic actions, large or small, can strengthen your connection with others and remind you of the positive impact you can have.

> Example : Participate in volunteering or offer your help to someone in need. These actions not only benefit others, but they can also give you a sense of accomplishment and gratitude for what you have.

2. Reinforce personal connections

Cultivating meaningful relationships with others can provide valuable emotional support and give meaning to your life. Deep connections with friends, family or support groups strengthen the sense of belonging and connection.

> Example : Spend time maintaining and deepening your relationships with important people in your life. Organize meetings, calls or activities to strengthen these links and remind you of the importance of these connections.

3. Celebrate contributions and achievements

Taking the time to celebrate your contributions and achievements can help you see the meaning and value of what you are doing. Recognizing your successes, big or small, brings you a sense of pride and gratitude.

> Example : After completing a project or achieving a goal, take a moment to recognize and celebrate your success. Whether by rewarding yourself or sharing your success with others, this recognition reinforces your sense of gratitude and accomplishment.

Finding meaning and cultivating gratitude are essential practices to transform sadness into an opportunity for growth and resilience. By seeking to understand the meaning of your experiences, by integrating gratitude into your daily life, and by developing resilience, you can navigate through difficult times with an enriching perspective. These practices not only help you overcome sadness, but they also give you the tools to create a more fulfilling and meaningful life.

Chapter 9: The art of letting go and accepting the ups and downs

Life is a series of ups and downs, and learning to let go and accept this fluctuation is essential to maintaining emotional well-being. This chapter explores how to embrace the impermanence of life, accept the varied emotions and find inner peace despite the turbulence.

9.1. The acceptance of impermanence

Impermanence is a fundamental reality of life. Everything is constantly changing, and accepting this truth can help you navigate more serenely through the ups and downs.

1. Understand the changing nature of life

Recognizing that situations, emotions and circumstances change is a crucial step towards acceptance. Accepting impermanence reduces resistance and finds serenity even when things do not go as planned.

> Example : When you are going through a difficult time, remember that pain and difficulties are temporary. By accepting this impermanence, you prepare to embrace the changes and see the light at the end of the tunnel.

2. Let go of rigid expectations

Rigid expectations can lead to frustration when things don't go as planned. Learning to let go and be flexible with your expectations allows you to better accept the ups and downs.

> Example : If a plan or objective does not come true as you had envisaged, adjust your expectations and be open to different results. This flexibility will help you navigate more easily through the changes.

3. Practice mindfulness of the present moment

Mindfulness helps you stay anchored in the present moment rather than focusing on past regrets or future anxieties. By focusing on the present moment, you can better accept emotional fluctuations and changing circumstances.

> Example : Devote a few minutes every day to the practice of mindfulness, whether through meditation or simply by paying attention to your feelings and your environment. This practice will help you stay centered despite the ups and downs.

9.2. Welcome varied emotions

Emotions are an integral part of the human experience. Learning to welcome and accept emotions, whether positive or negative, is essential to finding an emotional balance.

1. Avoid judging your emotions

Emotions are natural and should not be judged as good or bad. Learning to welcome all emotions, without judgment, allows you to live them fully and let them pass more easily.

> Example : When you feel a negative emotion such as sadness or anger, accept it without judgment. Observe this emotion without trying to suppress or change it, and allow yourself to feel it.

2. Use self-compassion to manage emotions

Self-compassion consists of treating your emotions with the same understanding and kindness that you would offer to a friend. It helps you accept and manage difficult emotions with gentleness and kindness.

> Example : When you face intense emotions, talk to yourself as you would with a person you like. Treat yourself to comforting words and understand that

emotions are part of the human experience.

3. Express emotions in a constructive way

Finding constructive ways to express and release emotions can help you manage them more effectively. This can include writing, art, or just talking to someone you trust.

> Example : Keep a diary to express your emotions, or engage in a creative activity such as painting or music. These methods can help you outsource your feelings and understand them better.

9.3. Find inner peace in the ups and downs

Inner peace is the ability to maintain a state of calm and serenity despite the fluctuations of life. Cultivating this inner peace allows you to navigate the ups and downs with a balanced and resilient attitude.

1. Practicing gratitude for the present

Gratitude helps you appreciate the present moment and find positive aspects even in times of difficulty. By focusing on what you are grateful for, you strengthen your inner peace.

> Example : Every day, write down three things you are grateful for. This practice can help you keep a positive perspective and appreciate the positive aspects of your life.

2. Cultivate relaxation and well-being habits

Incorporating relaxation habits into your daily routine can promote inner peace. These habits can include meditation, yoga, or moments of relaxation in nature.

> Example : Devotes time every day to relaxation activities, such as meditation or a walk in nature. These practices can help you reduce stress and find inner calm.

3. Adopt a mentality of letting go

Letting go is accepting what you can't control and focusing on what you can change. This mentality allows you to maintain inner peace even in the face of unforeseen or disconcerting circumstances.

> Example : When you are facing a situation beyond your control, focus on your own reactions and the aspects you can influence. By accepting what you cannot change, you reduce resistance and promote inner peace.

The art of letting go and accepting the ups and downs is essential to maintaining emotional balance and inner peace. By embracing the impermanence of life, welcoming all emotions without judgment, and cultivating relaxation and letting go practices, you can navigate more serenely through the challenges of life. This approach helps you find inner peace and remain resilient to the natural fluctuations of existence, by transforming the ups and downs into opportunities for growth and personal understanding.

Chapter 10: Take physical care of yourself for optimal well-being

Taking care of yourself physically is essential to maintain an emotional and mental balance. When you invest in your physical health, you create a solid foundation that supports not only your overall well-being, but also your resilience to emotional challenges. This chapter explores the key aspects of physical self-care and how these practices can strengthen your overall well-being.

10.1. The importance of a balanced diet

A balanced diet plays a crucial role in your physical and mental health. What you eat directly influences your energy level, your mood and your ability to manage stress.

1. Choose nutritious foods

Nutrient-rich foods, such as fruits, vegetables, lean proteins and whole grains, provide the energy and essentials necessary for your body and mind to function properly.

> Example : Include green vegetables, fresh fruits, nuts and lean proteins such as chicken or fish in your daily meals. These foods can help you maintain a stable energy level and a positive mood.

2. Avoid excesses and processed foods

Limiting the consumption of foods rich in added sugars, saturated fats and processed products can prevent energy fluctuations and negative impacts on your mental health.

> Example : Reduce the consumption of sugary drinks, fast food and foods rich in saturated fat. Instead, choose healthier alternatives, such as homemade smoothies and fruit or vegetable snacks.

3. Maintain adequate hydration

Hydration is essential for the proper functioning of your body and mind. Drinking enough water helps maintain your body function and improve your concentration and mood.

> Example : Aim to drink about 8 glasses of water a day, or more if you are active or if you live in a hot climate. Herbal infusions or flavored waters can also contribute to your hydration.

10.2. The importance of regular exercise

Regular exercise is a fundamental pillar of health and well-being. It not only improves your physical condition, but also your mental health by reducing stress and improving your mood.

1. Choose a physical activity that you like

Finding a form of exercise that you enjoy makes physical activity more enjoyable and sustainable. Whether it's walking, running, cycling, or yoga, the important thing is to choose an activity that you are motivated to practice regularly.

> Example : Explore different physical activities to discover the ones you like the most. For example, try dance, swimming, or fitness classes to find what suits you.

2. Establish a regular exercise routine

Creating a regular exercise routine allows you to reap consistent benefits for your physical and mental health. Even short but frequent sessions can have a significant impact.

> Example: Schedule 30-minute exercise sessions, 3 to 4 times a week. Include

cardiovascular exercises, muscle strengthening, and flexibility in your routine for complete well-being.

3. Listen to your body and avoid overwork

It is important to listen to your body and not overwork yourself. Give yourself days off and adjust your activity level according to your physical and mental state.

> Example : If you feel tired or pain, take days off or do lighter exercises such as walking or stretching. Listening to your body will help you prevent injuries and maintain a balanced exercise practice.

10.3. The role of sleep in physical and mental health

Quality sleep is crucial for general well-being. It influences your energy level, your concentration, and your ability to manage stress.

1. Establish a regular sleep routine

Going to bed and waking up at the same time every day helps regulate your circadian rhythm and improve the quality of your sleep. A regular routine promotes a restful rest.

> Example: Try to go to bed and wake up at the same time every day, even on weekends. Establish a relaxing routine before bed, such as reading a book or taking a hot bath.

2. Create a sleep-conducive environment

A comfortable and quiet sleeping environment contributes to a better sleep quality. Make sure your room is dark, fresh, and quiet.

> Example : Use blackout curtains, adjust the temperature of your room, and minimize noise. Also Consider relaxation techniques, such as deep breathing or

meditation, to help you fall asleep more easily.

3. Avoid stimulants before bedtime

Stimulants such as caffeine, nicotine and electronic screens can disturb your sleep. Avoid these stimulants in the hours before bedtime to promote restful sleep.

> Example : Limit caffeine consumption after the afternoon and avoid screens at least an hour before going to bed. Prefers relaxing activities such as reading or listening to soft music.

10.4. Listen to your body and practice self-care

Taking care of yourself also involves listening to your body and meeting its needs. Physical self-care includes stress management, self-care, and disease prevention.

1. Practicing stress management techniques

Chronic stress can have harmful effects on your physical health. Integrating stress management techniques, such as meditation, yoga, or breathing exercises, can help you maintain your physical and mental well-being.

> Example :Devote time every day to stress management techniques. Whether through meditation, yoga, or walks in nature, these practices can help reduce stress and improve your general well-being.

2. Take care of your personal hygiene

Maintaining good personal hygiene is important for your physical health. This includes regular care such as brushing teeth, skin care, and body hygiene.

> Example : Follow a daily personal care routine, such as brushing your teeth twice a day and skin care adapted to your skin type. These practices contribute to good hygiene and general well-being.

3. Perform regular health checks

Regular health checks can detect potential problems early and maintain good physical health. Be sure to consult a health professional regularly for preventive health check-ups.

> Example : Schedule regular visits to the doctor for health examinations and screenings. These checks are used to track your health and detect possible problems before they become serious.

Taking care of yourself physically is a fundamental aspect of general well-being. By adopting a balanced diet, practicing regular physical activity, ensuring quality sleep, and listening to your body's needs, you create a solid foundation for a healthy and fulfilling life. These physical care practices not only strengthen your physical health, but also your emotional resilience, allowing you to better manage life's challenges and promote overall well-being.

Chapter 11: Building a Positive and Hopeful Future

After going through a period of sadness, it is crucial to look to the future with a sense of hope and optimism. This chapter explores how to build a positive future by setting goals, establishing healthy routines, and cultivating a growth mindset.

11.1. Set meaningful goals

Setting clear and meaningful goals can provide direction and motivation during difficult times. Goals give you something to work towards and help you move forward despite the sadness.

1. Define short- and long-term objectives

Short-term goals are immediate steps that you can achieve quickly, while long-term goals represent broader aspirations. Setting both types of goals can offer a balance between immediate success and a broader vision of the future.

Example: Set short-term goals such as following a new activity or learning a skill. At the same time, set long-term goals related to your personal or professional aspirations.

2. Create a detailed action plan

A well-defined action plan helps you break down your objectives into concrete and manageable steps. Identify the resources you need, set deadlines, and plan the steps necessary to achieve your goals.

Example: If your goal is to start a new career, create a plan detailing the steps to follow, such as searching for training, updating your resume, and finding networking opportunities.

3. Track progress and celebrate successes

Regularly evaluate your progress and celebrate successes, even the little ones, strengthens your motivation and your sense of accomplishment. Celebrating the steps reached reminds you that you are moving towards your goals.

Example: Use a journal or an application to track your progress. Every time you reach an important milestone, take the time to celebrate it and recognize your efforts.

11.2. Establish healthy routines

Healthy routines can contribute to your overall well-being and your ability to face challenges. By establishing positive habits, you create an environment that supports growth and resilience.

1. Create a balanced daily routine

A balanced routine includes aspects such as sleep, diet, exercise and leisure time. Be sure to integrate these elements into your daily life to maintain your physical and emotional well-being.

Example: Establish a daily routine that includes a regular bedtime, balanced meals, and time for exercise. Also includes moments to relax and enjoy activities you enjoy.

2. Incorporate well-being practices

Wellness practices, such as meditation, mindfulness, and relaxing activities, can help manage stress and improve your state of mind. Integrate these practices into your routine to promote a sense of calm and clarity.

Example: Devote a few minutes each day to meditation or mindfulness. Use applications or guided techniques to help you develop these practices.

3. Maintain a work-life balance

Ensuring a healthy work-life balance is essential to avoid excessive stress and preserve your well-being. Establish clear boundaries between your professional responsibilities and your personal time.

Example: Set regular working hours and respect them. Also plan personal activities and moments of relaxation to maintain balance.

11.3. Cultivating a growth mindset

Adopting a growth mindset means believing in your ability to evolve, learn and adapt. This mentality allows you to see challenges as opportunities for learning and personal development.

1. Welcoming challenges as opportunities

A growth mindset allows you to see obstacles as opportunities to grow rather than failures. Welcoming challenges with a positive attitude can strengthen your resilience and motivation.

Example: When you face a challenge, ask yourself what you can learn from this situation. Adopt an attitude of curiosity and openness in the face of difficulties.

2. Encourage continuous learning

Continuous learning allows you to develop new skills and adapt to changes. Constantly look for ways to learn and improve yourself, whether through formal studies, readings or practical experiences.

Example: Register for a course or workshop in a field that interests you. Read books or articles on topics that you are passionate about to expand your knowledge.

3. Practice self-compassion and patience

The practice of self-compassion and patience is essential to maintain a growth mentality. Be kind to yourself when you face difficulties and give yourself the time you need to progress.

Example : When you encounter obstacles or mistakes, treat yourself with kindness and understanding. Recognize that growth takes time and that each step is part of your journey.

Building a positive and hopeful future involves setting meaningful goals, establishing healthy routines, and cultivating a growth mindset. By setting clear goals, integrating wellness practices into your daily life, and adopting a positive attitude towards challenges, you can create a solid foundation for a fulfilling future. These practices will help you navigate through difficult times with hope and determination, paving the way for a life filled with opportunities and personal growth.

At the end of this journey through the pages of this book, it is essential to remember that the search for well-being is a continuous process, not a final destination. Taking care of yourself, accepting the ups and downs of life, and building a positive future are efforts that require patience, perseverance and self-bevolence.

Each chapter of this book has been designed to give you tools and perspectives to navigate through challenges and promote a fulfilling life. Whether you seek to understand and embrace the impermanence of life, adopt physical care practices, or cultivate a growth mentality, it is important to remember that every small step counts.

1. The acceptance of impermanence invites you to understand that ups and downs are an integral part of human existence. Accepting this constant flow of change allows you to live more serenely and find stability in change.

2. The welcome of varied emotions encourages you to fully live each emotion

without judgment, using self-compassion and constructive expression to navigate through emotional challenges with a balanced attitude.

3. Taking care of yourself physically highlights the importance of a balanced diet, regular physical activity, and quality sleep to support your general well-being and strengthen your resilience.

As you put these principles into practice, remember that the journey to well-being is personal and unique to everyone. There is no single path or universal solutions, but by integrating these practices into your daily life, you build a solid foundation for a more serene and fulfilled existence.

Never forget that every day is a new opportunity to get closer to your best self. Welcome challenges as opportunities for growth, celebrate your successes, and be kind to yourself throughout this journey.

Thank you for getting involved in this exploration towards well-being. May you find inner peace, strength and joy over your days, while keeping in mind that well-being is a continuous journey, made of discoveries and growth.

My sincere greetings and wishes for well-being,

GERALD B.K

www.ingramcontent.com/pod-product-compliance
Lightning Source LLC
Chambersburg PA
CBHW070146230526
45471CB00002B/538

"Life is not to wait for the storm to pass, but to learn to dance in the rain."

- Vivian Greene